Contents

About the authors

Richard Lewis is a Senior Fellow in Health Policy at the King's Fund. He carries out policy analysis and research, with a special interest in foundation trusts, commissioning, US managed care, patient safety and primary care. He is also an independent health care consultant. He has a background in health service management, and spent several years as executive director of a large health authority in south-west London. Richard has a PhD in health policy.

Jennifer Dixon is Director of Policy at the King's Fund. She has researched and written widely on health care reform in the United Kingdom and internationally. Her background is in clinical medicine and policy analysis, and she has a PhD in health services research. She was Harkness Fellow in New York in 1990, and Policy Advisor to the Chief Executive of the National Health Service between 1998 and 2000. Jennifer is currently a board member of both the Audit Commission and the Healthcare Commission.

Introduction

The government is currently engaged in a programme of rapid reform of the National Health Service (NHS). The aims of these reforms include ensuring rapid access to and greater responsiveness of services; delivering more services in a community setting; making more effort to 'manage demand' for NHS care effectively (that is, to plan care and contain escalating health care costs); and reducing health inequalities. This paper examines the role and contribution expected of primary care in delivering these aims.

The term 'primary care' is used relatively loosely in the NHS. It commonly refers to family doctors and their teams. However, it also refers to a wide array of professionals such as pharmacists and dentists, as well as to the commissioning organisations – primary care trusts (PCTs) – that are responsible for overseeing local NHS services. In this paper we use the term to refer to general practice-based and community nursing services and PCTs.

The government's chosen approach to delivering change within the NHS is increasingly reliant on the introduction of market mechanisms. Primary care will play a vital role in the creation of this market approach – both because market incentives will be strengthened in primary care itself and because primary care teams will play an important role in applying market incentives to other parts of the health system.

Primary care will be particularly central to any strategy to manage demand – something that is increasingly preoccupying the NHS as budgets run out, despite record increases in resources (Lewis and Dixon

2005). There are several reasons for this central position. The generalist role of the GP and the long-term relationships that are often formed with patients give the primary care team a unique view of the performance of the health system as a whole. In addition, the delivery of primary care is intimately related to the delivery of specialist services; what GPs and primary care teams do in their surgeries impacts on the role of and demand for hosital care. Therefore, the 'commissioning' of much hospital care is a reflection of the practice of primary care.

The primary care sector – for so long the most stable and enduring part of the NHS – has been undergoing a sustained, if quiet, revolution since the 1990s. This revolution has seen the ending of the monopoly over provision of independently contracted GPs, a radical change in access to first contact care, a raft of new targets and, latterly, a renewed interest in general practice-based commissioning. Now, primary care is set for more change, with a White Paper due in early 2006 and a commitment already in place to structural reforms that include the rapid introduction of 'practice-based commissioning', new strategic commissioning roles for a reduced number of PCTs, and the longer-term divestment by PCTs of their responsibilities as community health service providers in favour of a mixed and contestable (that is, subject to competition) market (Crisp 2005).

Whatever the merits of this rapid and substantive programme of reform, it is clear that there are obvious strengths and weaknesses in primary care at present, which will have an impact on the degree to which the government is successful in its aims. With respect to provision, on the one hand, public satisfaction with family doctors and care by general practices is consistently high (Healthcare Commission 2004; 2005). Furthermore, GPs have recently achieved 92 per cent of the wide range of quality targets under their new contract. On the other hand, the quality of primary care (although on average high) is variable on a practice-by-practice basis, and quality has been poor, particularly in parts of some inner cities, for some decades (London Health Planning

Consortium 1981). However, there have been only limited ways of identifying and addressing poor practice available to PCTs and their predecessor bodies.

With respect to commissioning, the prevailing consensus is that this activity is underdeveloped in PCTs; this needs to change urgently if commissioners are going to provide an adequate counterweight to new incentives for acute and foundation trusts to admit patients (such as the new NHS 'payment by results' system) and for foundation trusts to meet the exacting financial requirements set by Monitor (the independent regulator of NHS foundation trusts).

Recent policy developments

In 1997 the introduction of personal medical service (PMS) pilots marked a radical departure for general practice (Lewis *et al* 2001). New types of organisations (both public and private) were able to contract to provide primary care and new services that responded to the very specific needs of different types of patient group. In addition, a new cadre of salaried, rather than independently contracted, GPs developed. Currently, 37 per cent of practitioners offer primary care under PMS arrangements (Department of Health 2005a).

By 2003 a new national contract for general medical services (GMS) had also been negotiated. This contract replaced many of the existing fees and allowances, with a new capitation (per head) payment, together with quality payments linked to a comprehensive set of standards.

These two contractual changes have ushered in a very new world for family doctors and their teams and given PCTs far greater power to shape local services than hitherto. It can be argued that, for the first time, local NHS organisations can directly commission primary care (although the ability to exercise these new powers has been hampered by a lack of PCT capacity). At the same time, the government has been at pains to increase access for patients to alternative sources of primary care. Walk-in centres, NHS Direct and new commuter surgeries have all been developed. These have proved popular with patients, with nearly 16 million people accessing NHS Direct online or by telephone each year and two million patients visiting walk-in centres (Department of Health 2005b). As a consequence of these policies, patients are increasingly able to access primary care from a variety of sources.

The commissioning function has also undergone rapid change. PCTs in England now handle about 85 per cent of the revenue budget of the

NHS, commissioning primary, intermediate and secondary care. Soon they will all be broadly co-terminous with local authorities, and new flexibilities will allow budgets to be pooled across sectors to tackle joint problems. Primary care clinicians, through their majority on the Professional Executive Committee (PEC) of the PCT, are intended, in theory at least, to set strategy and act as the 'engine room' of the organisation (NHS Executive 1999). However, recent government policy has highlighted the potential gains to be made from the devolution of commissioning to general practice level (Department of Health 2004) and, from 1 April 2005, all practices have had the right to commission care for their registered patients using an 'indicative budget' (that is, commissioning resources remain formally under the control of the PCT, but power to allocate these resources is passed to practices).

The combination of the new contractual flexibilities and commissioning incentives is likely to result in innovations in both the provision and the commissioning of care. New providers will increasingly enter the primary care market (under 'alternative provider medical services', 'specialist PMS' and new GMS contracts). It seems likely that an increasing number will be from the independent sector or from NHS hospital or foundation trusts. Some will offer comprehensive care, whereas others ('third party providers') may offer only niche services such as chronic disease management or urgent and out-of-hours care services. Recent guidance has emphasised the requirement to offer contestable community health services and instructs PCTs to divest themselves of provider responsibilities in all but exceptional circumstances (Crisp 2005).

The policy to encourage practices to hold budgets was developed partly to engage more clinicians in commissioning in the hope that they would contain health care costs. The ability of practices to hold commissioning budgets provides an opportunity for an expansion of community-based services. Practice-based commissioners (PBCs) will face the classic 'make or buy' business decision and may increasingly choose to provide services in-house (or contract with new providers) rather than continuing to refer to established hospitals. As in the past, commissioners currently face obstacles in transferring care out of hospital because only marginal, not full, costs are released by providers and there are only weak incentives for commissioners to seek to prevent avoidable admissions – for example, with respect to care of patients with long-term conditions. Both of these obstacles are likely to disappear once payment by results has been implemented across the NHS.

What are the main problems and challenges?

Notwithstanding significant recent developments in primary care policy, a number of problems remain.

Provision

- A lack of choice of GP remains a persistent problem in areas of England such as London, or where geography makes choice more difficult to achieve (Audit Commission 2004).

- There is variable quality of provision of primary care, with poor care in some areas, particularly inner cities.

- Much care remains ad hoc and reactive, although the new GP contract now incentivises systematic, proactive and managed care for selected conditions.

- There is an inadequate focus on primary and secondary prevention of ill-health.

- There are relatively few mechanisms to improve poor-quality practice such as peer review, performance-related financial incentives or, ultimately, loss of contract to provide.

- Although the problems with immediate access to primary care services have eased with the successful application of the 24–48 hour target, primary care is still struggling in some areas to meet the levels of responsiveness required, particularly in relation to the working population (Healthcare Commission 2005).

Commissioning

■ There is little evidence that commissioning in the NHS has made a significant or strategic impact on secondary care services (Smith *et al* 2004). Nor have sophisticated commissioning skills been developed uniformly with PCTs, despite the strong likelihood that current financial incentives in the NHS encourage acute trusts to increase admissions.

■ Through payment by results there are stronger incentives for commissioners to improve primary, community and social services so that the risk of costly treatment in hospital is reduced. The ability of PCTs to identify effective low-cost options for care is, however, very weak (Evans 2005).

■ There are few incentives for PCTs or practices in their role as commissioner to be responsive to patients as consumers.

■ Many PCTs have struggled to engage local primary care clinicians effectively (Regan 2002; NHS Alliance/Primary Care Report 2003).

■ There are weak incentives to encourage large-scale take-up of practice-based commissioning, especially where the PCT is currently in deficit. This is particularly pertinent given the new government target to universalise practice-based commissioning by the end of 2006. Evidence from previous incarnations of practice-based commissioning suggests that it has some potential to manage demand for secondary care and to encourage changes in clinical practice in primary care (Lewis 2004; Smith *et al* 2004).

What should be done?
Three challenges

A major challenge for the government must be to boost commissioning, while at the same time managing financial instability in the acute sector. If this is not done, there is every chance that the current mix of financial incentives will lead to acute trusts maximising income and PCTs being too weak to counter the inevitable flow of resources into the acute sector. This may result in the ad hoc loss of community-based services and suboptimal distribution of health resources.

The current reforms imply new roles for both PBCs and PCTs (*see* box, below).

NEW ROLES FOR PRIMARY CARE TRUSTS (PCTS) AND PRACTICE-BASED COMMISSIONERS (PBCS)

PCT roles
- improving the health of the community and reducing health inequalities
- securing the provision of safe, high-quality services
- providing contract management on behalf of their practices and the public
- engaging with local people and other local service providers to hear patients' views and provide coherent access to health and social care
- acting as providers of services only where it is not possible to have separate providers
- emergency planning

continued overleaf

NEW ROLES FOR PRIMARY CARE TRUSTS (PCTS) AND PRACTICE-BASED COMMISSIONERS (PBCS) *continued*

PBC roles
- designing improved patient pathways
- working in partnership with PCTs to creat convenient community-based services
- taking responsibility for a budget delegated from the PCT covering acute, community and emergency care
- managing the budget effectively

Source: Adapted from Crisp (2005)

A central issue is whether current structures and incentives within the NHS are broadly appropriate and sufficient to engineer a substantial improvement in the quality of primary care and commissioning over the next few years. It is currently the case that the development of these functions is not as important in the overall assessment of PCTs' performance by strategic health authorities as their ability to meet hospital-related targets. This fact is likely to have inhibited a local focus on these issues. This could change if the Department of Health increases the priority of this part of the NHS agenda relative to other, hitherto dominant, priorities. The forthcoming White Paper on care out of hospital is an opportunity for this shift in priorities to occur.

However, it is our view that current opportunities to develop both commissioning and provision of primary care have failed to generate sufficient motivation for change. Notwithstanding any further prioritisation of these issues, more radical solutions should at least be considered (although such solutions come with risks attached).

Below we consider the ways in which three key challenges facing primary care and commissioning might be addressed.

Challenge 1: Quality of primary care

The first challenge is how to improve the quality of primary care, particularly in inner city areas. One way could be to encourage greater choice of primary care provider and offer larger rewards to providers who attract more patients, subject to meeting quality standards. Current policies are beginning to address the choice issue, mainly through the central and local procurement of alternative types of care (such as walk-in centres and new practices in under-served areas) and by giving more powers to PCTs to commission primary care. However, these measures, although welcome, will not deliver change that is either substantial or rapid enough. Higher-powered incentives are required and a number of new initiatives might be considered.

Should patients be able to 'pick and choose' primary care services?

Radical options for increasing the responsiveness of primary care for patients have been mooted. These focus primarily on separating out different elements of the primary care contract, opening each to competition. One suggestion is that of 'split registration', where patients may register for services at more than one practice (for example, for patients who want access to a primary care provider near the workplace). More radical still would be the introduction of payment by results for primary care. Under this system, patient registration would cease and primary care teams would receive specific payments for seeing and treating patients. Income would depend on services provided, rather than mainly on an annual capitation payment per patient registered. This system could operate with or without patient registration. If the latter course were chosen, patients would in theory be allowed to receive primary care services anywhere, as is the case in some other countries.

The case for this sort of change is supported by the fact that patients already appear to be satisfied with new types of direct access primary care such as NHS Direct and walk-in centres (although their value for money might be questioned as they appear to add additional services rather than substitute for existing ones). However, these additional forms of access do not undermine the principle that a patient should register with a single primary care team – a hallmark of NHS primary care. Registration has significant benefits and there would probably be serious drawbacks if it were to be scrapped, for example, by pursuing the options outlined above.

Patient registration underpins the continuity of relationships between patients and their primary carers. It also supports a public health approach and ensures that there is clear clinical responsibility for care management, particularly important in the overall management of long-term conditions. As important is the evidence that interpersonal continuity is associated with better health outcomes and lower costs (Saultz and Lochner 2005). Although the electronic patient record offers the possibility of continuity of summary clinical information across a large number of clinicians, this does not replace the human clinician–patient relationship that can build up over time. This is likely to be particularly important for patients with long-standing and complex medical conditions – a group that currently incur significant NHS expenditure. Even split registration would raise difficulties, for example, in assigning overall clinical responsibility and managing practice-level commissioning budgets.

Moreover, fragmentation of the primary care contract, for example, through a solely fee-for-service system, could increase costs because practices would have clear financial incentives to encourage access. This is similar to the increase in demand and supply of NHS dentistry after the introduction of 'piece rates' following the 1990 contract. It would seem therefore that the registration of patients with a single practice should probably continue.

Should greater contestability be introduced?
Aside from the issue of patient registration, there remains a need to address the deficits in provision identified earlier (*see* Provision, p 7).

This is particularly the case in inner city areas where variable quality is combined with a current undersupply of services.

The government has begun a programme of national procurement of primary care for areas with poor access. However, a more radical approach, and one that sits more comfortably with the commitment to decentralisation, might be to experiment with an 'open market' for primary care. In particular, this might serve to address 'anti-competitive' behaviours – such as selective closures of doctors' lists and strictly defined catchment areas. Although PCTs currently enjoy the power to let new primary care contracts, including to the independent sector (and have had these powers since 1997), in practice, few additional contracts have been let. Where they have, these have generally been to traditional GP-owned and -managed organisations.

In an open market, any appropriately qualified professional (or organisation employing qualified professionals) would have the right to contract for services and register patients, subject to the same performance-management and quality-assurance framework as other local providers. This may increase the supply of, and therefore the competition between, primary care providers. In particular, it may encourage a greater involvement of private sector providers by removing regulatory and cultural barriers to their entry. Such competition, it can be argued, may increase the responsiveness of primary care services to patient needs and may overcome the apparent current inertia to commissioning primary care more actively. More patient choice would challenge the oft-cited criticism that primary care operates as a cartel in which doctors choose patients rather than the other way around.

Such a radical approach also comes with risks attached. Open lists for general practice teams may reallocate the current, already scarce, workforce away from more challenging populations (arguably with a greater need for primary care). It may also serve to decrease profitability of practices in other geographical areas, leading to instability and greater incentives to 'cherry pick' less needy patients. Lastly, it could be argued that greater competition between primary care providers will inhibit their willingness to co-operate in the sharing of good clinical practice and the development of broader local health strategy.

These risks might be mitigated, however. For example, the current capitation formula (which already provides additional remuneration for populations with higher needs) could be used to provide additional financial incentives to encourage practice in poorly served areas. Any move towards a more contestable primary care sector would require careful regulation, in particular, to ensure no loss of equity or quality. However, the extent of the workforce shortage in primary care should not be underestimated and may form a brake to future reform.

An alternative to an open market for primary care (which relies on patients to drive up quality through their choice of primary care team) is greater power for PCTs to remove the contracts of providers that are not delivering a good enough quality of care. Currently, most existing practices enjoy a secure tenure and essentially 'preferred provider' status. There is currently ambiguity as to whether failure to meet quality standards set out in the Quality and Outcomes Framework (this provides incentives to improve quality and is a voluntary part of the GP contract) is sufficient grounds for contract removal. In future, there may be a case for the periodic market testing of all primary care contractors. In this way, contracts could be renewed or terminated on the basis of whether or not other bidding contractors could offer a better service.

The government has also announced that contestability in community health services is to be introduced following the divestment of provider services by PCTs. This policy is designed to increase patient choice and the responsiveness of services to the needs of different individuals. However, such a policy will require careful thought if it is to be implemented successfully. The government has yet to spell out what its vision of a contestable market is. Simply transferring PCT provider services to another provider would replace one monopoly with another. Breaking up a single PCT provider into several smaller organisations might generate competition but potentially at higher cost and perhaps causing difficulties with professional training and development.

Moreover, there are no ready structures available to which community services might migrate. Some nursing services may sit comfortably as part of general practice teams and the integration of general practice and community nursing services has been a long-standing goal of some providers for many years. This type of integration contradicts the notion of choice and contestability. If anything, patients would experience less choice under this arrangement as their community nursing service would be determined solely by their choice of GP (although they might receive very high-quality care). If choice is to be experienced by patients, new capacity will be needed.

As community services leave the ambit of PCTs, there is the possibility for a new type of provider organisation to emerge – the public benefit organisation accountable to local communities. With support, PCT provider services could be transformed into a range of socially owned and controlled, not-for-profit companies that can build patient and community empowerment into their core purpose. These arrangements would loosely mirror the governance arrangements in foundation trusts. Arguably, communities will have more reason to engage with community providers, with whom they are likely to have a long-term relationship, than with hospitals. Clearly the government also envisages a role for not-for-profit companies and it would be interesting to assess which type of provider organisation is optimal.

Challenge 2: Commissioning

The second and very major challenge is how to invigorate the commissioning function (*see* box, below) and redress the imbalance of power in relation to NHS hospital providers.

WHAT IS COMMISSIONING?

Elements of commissioning functions

Planning
- determining priorities
- identifying need
- identifying providers and capacity
- assessing budgetary need

Purchasing
- deciding which services are contracted out
- identifying which providers to use
- designing and negotiating contracts
- putting governance arrangements in place

Monitoring
- monitoring delivery and activity volumes
- assessing clinical quality
- assessing patient satisfaction

Source: Adapted from Bramley-Harker and Lewis (2005)

The current government response is to develop the strength of the commissioning function through a number of related strategies, for example:
- fewer and bigger PCTs and the combination of a number of essential functions (such as the procurement of services) across more than one PCT

- greater engagement of physicians through practice-based commissioning
- stronger performance management and benchmarking of PCTs against a strict set of criteria, combined with regulation
- better investment in training staff, assessing the competence of PCTs and improving the commissioning infrastructure (for example, through information systems for tracking activity and cost).

However, whether these strategies will be sufficient is a moot point given the scale of the task in hand. Again, more radical options may need to be considered and perhaps piloted.

Practice-based commissioning offers promise in its ability to add bite to the commissioning function, in particular, by improving the identification of need, designing appropriate care pathways that offer a smooth and rational transition across organisational boundaries, and monitoring the quality of delivery. However, as discussed above, the current incentives on offer may be too weak to overcome the entrenched culture among GPs of resisting a role in demand management or to stimulate the scale of change required. Instead, negotiating 'real' budgets with PBCs, whereby any savings are accrued as profits (and conversely overspends are managed as losses), may serve to increase the impact of this initiative. Private sector organisations may feel more comfortable than groups of independently contracted GPs in holding this sort of financial risk. However, GP practices are already beginning to form clusters, thereby creating the potential for more powerful local commissioning agencies with the confidence and management skills to take on financial risk.

Notwithstanding the scope for using hard-edged financial incentives to stimulate change, the incentive effect of endowing clinicians with the power simply to innovate should not be underestimated. Therefore, a combination of financial and non-financial incentives may achieve a significant stimulus for change.

The role of contestability to increase the power and performance of commissioning also offers intriguing possibilities, although it carries potential risks. Contestability could in theory be applied to the strategic organisations that oversee practice-based commissioning (PCTs), to the management that supports practice-based commissioning and to PBCs themselves. The forms of contestability might include the following:

- competition between commissioning organisations for NHS-let contracts
- competition between commissioning management organisations for contracts let by large medical groups (of primary and possibly secondary care physicians)
- competition between commissioners for patients.

The King's Fund, following research on managed care organisations in the USA, has suggested that some competitive forces might be applied to PCTs (such as the periodic tendering of management support) (Dixon *et al* 2004). Such contestability is feasible (and indeed at least one example is already being explored within the NHS (Donnelly 2005)). Arguably, such arrangements would keep management on their toes for fear of losing the contract. Of course, all managers recognise that poor performance in their job could result in their dismissal, but periodic tendering means that the incumbent management would need to demonstrate that their performance was better than that of a potential alternative, rather than simply avoiding an obvious organisational failure.

For their part, PCTs must have the ability to deal effectively with practices where the performance as commissioner is below an acceptable standard. Currently, the government has indicated that all GP practices are expected to operate as PBCs. However, it is likely that at least some will struggle. In some cases, they will simply fail to innovate, offering only traditional services to their patients, but in other cases a 'failure' in commissioning may mean a significant overspending of the allocated budget. Although there is considerable complexity involved in setting a 'fair' budget for a relatively small population served by a practice, there will undoubtedly be cases where an overspend by a PBC represents an overuse of scarce resources, thus depriving other practices' patients, and possibly poor clinical management.

Currently, commissioning responsibilities are not core activities governed by the primary care contract. Therefore, PCTs may find it hard to deal with substandard commissioning effectively. Although PBCs may be stripped of their rights to commission (with the budget transferred to another practice or commissioning agency), this may not resolve the problem if clinical practice does not change. Ultimately, commissioning should be seen as an essential role of any organisation contracting to provide primary care and regulated through greater powers for PCTs in the giving and taking away of contracts.

In some areas, groups of GPs are joining together to employ managers to help them manage practice-based commissioning across groups of practices (sometimes, but not always, forming geographical localities). Here, it could be argued that management is contestable; this has the advantage that the clinical staff select management to facilitate commissioning, not the other way around. It is also the physicians who decide whether continuity with a group of managers is worthwhile, rather than the current state of affairs within PCTs where clinicians and PCT managers are wedded together.

As practice-based commissioning rolls out, there are new opportunities for independent management groups to develop and offer services to PBCs. These management teams could compete with each other, based on their commissioning skills – for example, their ability to stratify patients by clinical risk or develop innovative clinical pathways. As PCTs becoming rightly more demanding of their PBCs over time, the demand for expert commissioning management may increase.

A further form of contestability is to allow patients to choose their commissioner. Of course, the current rights of patients to choose their

GP (albeit limited in many areas), together with practice-based commissioning, imply that, in effect, patients will soon be able to exercise this choice. As practice-based commissioning develops, patients may well factor into their decision some notion of the overall package of care that they wish to receive – practices will offer different ranges of services in their own surgeries and will vary in the way in which, and from whom, they commission those services that they do not provide. Clearly, if this were to happen, there would need to be far more information available to patients to inform their choice.

It is also clear, however, that the clustering of practices into commissioning groups may serve to restrict patients' ability to have a meaningful choice of commissioner – in some areas all local practices may offer very similar approaches to commissioning, all co-ordinated by a collective management structure. This may be desirable on the grounds of quality and interprofessional collaboration, but it is scarcely consistent with patient choice.

Patients' choice of commissioner could be enhanced by the purposeful design of a 'commissioning market'. This market would go beyond a choice of PBC to that of a choice of PCT or conglomerate of commissioning practices not defined geographically, but defined by patient enrolees. By looking to the USA, a number of potential models for achieving this change become apparent.

The growth of managed-care organisations is underpinned by competition between them for enrolees. This form of competition can be a source of motivation for quality improvement, as we have already said. In an English context, groups of primary care teams and strategic commissioning bodies (currently PCTs) could be formed. These new integrated alliances would compete with each other for patients and would share a mutual dependency that could strengthen the collaboration between commissioning managers and clinicians. They would be subject to assessment by an independent regulator and would not necessarily serve a population tightly defined by geography (indeed there would have to be overlap between these groups if competition were to thrive). Physicians could work exclusively for a particular commissioner, or for more than one, giving patients a choice of strategic commissioner.

There are of course potential pitfalls associated with all of these ideas for increasing contestability. For example, the loss of a geographical focus to commissioning (such as might be created if PCTs were to become contestable or if groups of PBCs served non-contiguous populations) might make it more difficult for services to be provided equitably, for public health to be delivered, and for there to be appropriate integration between health and local authority services such as social care. In addition, greater competition for patients and pressure to be efficient might encourage commissioners to attract a disproportionate number of healthy patients over those with pre-existing conditions. This potential for 'cream skimming' would need to be heavily regulated. Furthermore, competition between PCT–practice alliances would require such a market to be created from scratch – a potentially onerous undertaking – and by definition would involve the duplication of scarce commissioning skills.

While the ideas above are designed to improve the power of commissioners, it is important to note that, whatever mechanism is selected, there is an urgent need to invest in commissioning skills. These skills will, in part at least, include advanced data analysis, which is necessary for understanding patterns of current and future demand. In turn, it is vital that commissioners are supported by information systems that provide rapid and accurate data. Currently, the NHS is relatively lacking in all of these respects. In addition, there is a need to develop an appropriate framework to judge the success or otherwise of commissioners. Clearly, the ability to remain within budgetary constraints is one measure of success, however, other indicators of performance are required to offer a more sophisticated appraisal.

Challenge 3: Clinical integration

The third main challenge is to find a better way of integrating primary and secondary care, in particular, to meet the increasing cost of health care for people with multiple and chronic conditions. The Department of Health has identified as a priority the need to ensure that specialist care must be provided within a 'planned network' incorporating all providers (NHS and non-NHS) within a geographical area. However, this planning must take place within an environment that fosters competition between those same providers (Department of Health 2005c).

The NHS in England has been characterised by external commentators as suffering from an 'iron curtain' dividing primary and secondary care (Wiener et al 2001). The greater cohesion and partnership between primary care physicians and specialists in some US managed-care organisations has been noted and seen as beneficial, not least in the care of long-term conditions (Dixon et al 2004). The promising developments under 'PMS Plus' to integrate primary and secondary care need to accelerate. Other policies, such as the introduction of an independent sector to primary care and the existence of foundation trusts, may accelerate this trend through a greater availability of capital investment for new community-based specialist facilities.

Great interest has been shown within the NHS in the 'Kaiser model' of integrated care (based on the US managed-care organisation Kaiser Permanente, where primary and secondary care clinicians co-exist within a single medical group, sharing the same clinical priorities and financial incentives). A critical message about Kaiser is, however, that this type of integration occurs within the overall context of a fiercely competitive environment among managed-care organisations. Without the nudge from competition, the worry would be that large integrated monopolies would develop, with few incentives to improve performance or to be responsive to patients.

As discussed above, the creation of this environment may not be suitable for the NHS in England, or certainly not at this stage before competition is sufficiently developed. The Department of Health, or a new economic regulator, would need to consider this issue if NHS foundation trusts were to seek to buy up or provide community services and primary care.

The Kaiser approach would mean significant change in NHS structures and culture, with the creation of new, cohesive and independent medical organisations formally separated from hospital infrastructure and with an 'insurance plan' attached.

However, such a model could be anglicised and more modest. Effective, developments could be initiated in the shape of multi-specialty groups (including primary care physicians) or networks. Practice-based commissioning, in theory at least, offers the right incentives for this to happen.

PBCs now have the power to determine what skill mix they require within their core team to manage care cost effectively and to fund this using their unified budget (subject to an appropriate financial governance arrangement). This may well lead to primary care teams expanding to incorporate a range of specialist practitioners (for example, diagnosticians or consultants in major outpatient specialties), allowing more care to be retained within the primary care setting. By bringing generalists and specialists together in the same team, a more integrated view of clinical priorities for investment might be obtained than is the case currently – particularly if all clinicians shared the same financial incentives related to their management of overall resources.

Conclusion

This paper briefly considers the challenges that face primary care provision and the commissioning function within the NHS. These two agendas are inter-related. Urgent action is required if the unfolding of powerful incentives applied to acute hospital advisers is not to overwhelm the NHS. A strong commissioning function, rooted in the effective delivery of primary care, is needed to act as a counterbalance.

There is a range of approaches that may be taken to address these challenges. Some, such as strengthened incentives for PBCs, simply build on what is currently in place. Others offer a more radical vision. In particular, the role of markets and patient choice as a driver for quality improvement may have a place.

In an earlier paper, we recognised that the NHS faces a number of objectives – among them greater efficiency, higher quality and greater equity (Lewis and Dixon 2005). These policy goals are likely to be in tension at certain times and inevitably there will be trade-offs between them.

Contestability may drive up efficiency but perhaps at the expense of interprofessional and interorganisational collaboration – such collaboration often being a prerequisite for high-quality services. Clinical integration is likely to be more easily achieved if supported by stable relationships between organisations (or even the formal integration of organisations along a care pathway). However, contestability and choice rely on separation and competition between different components of the health care system. Already we see a growth in clusters of PBCs where a collaborative mode of working lessens the potential for competition within primary care. Similarly, there is perhaps an irony that the better integration of primary and secondary care, an overt policy goal for more than a decade and now a possibility if foundation trusts were to extend into primary care, may now be seen to be the enemy of the new objective of contestability. Clearly, these tensions will not be easily resolved.

The debate over NHS reform goes beyond a search for the right structural fit. Ultimately, the discussion is as much about notions of what sort of incentives will best drive quality improvement and efficiency. Much of the recent debate has focused on the greater use of financial incentives. But there is evidence that financial incentives may crowd out more 'intrinsic' incentives such as professionalism and altruism (Marshall and Harrison 2005) and therefore they should be used with care. Clearly, getting the right blend between financial and other incentives to achieve the optimal outcome is a complex undertaking.

If greater use of market-style mechanisms in primary care is inevitable, as government pronouncements suggest that it is, then careful regulation will be required if service quality, patient safety and equity are all to be maintained. This subject will be explored in the next paper in the 'NHS Market Futures' series (Dixon 2005).

References

Audit Commission (2004). *Transforming Primary Care: The role of PCTs in shaping and supporting general practice*. London: Audit Commission.

Bramley-Harker E, Lewis D (2005). *Commissioning in the NHS: Challenges and opportunities*. London: NERA Economic Consulting.

Crisp N (2005). *Commissioning a Patient-led NHS*. London: Department of Health.

Department of Health (2005a). *Statistics for General Medical Practitioners in England 1994–2004*. London: Department of Health.

Department of Health (2005b). *Chief Executive's Report to the NHS*. London: Department of Health.

Department of Health (2005c). *Creating a Patient-led NHS: Delivering the NHS Improvement Plan*. London: Department of Health.

Department of Health (2004). *Practice Based Commissioning: Engaging practices in commissioning*. London: Department of Health.

Dixon J (2005). *Regulation in the New NHS Market*. London: King's Fund, in press.

Dixon J, Lewis R, Rosen R, Gray D and Finlayson B (2004). *Managing Chronic Disease: What can we learn from the US experience?* London: King's Fund.

Donnelly L (2005). 'Oxford commissioning to be outsourced', *Health Service Journal*, 13 October 2005.

Evans D (2005). *Developing a Business for Chronic Disease Management*. London: King's Fund, in press.

Healthcare Commission (2005). *Patient Survey: Primary care trust*. London: Healthcare Commission.

Healthcare Commission (2004). *Patient Survey Report 2004: Primary care*. London: Healthcare Commission.

Lewis R (2004). *Practice-led Commissioning: Harnessing the power of the primary care frontline*. London: King's Fund. Available at: www.kingsfund.org.uk/pdf/practiceledcommissioning.pdf (accessed on 3 November 2005).

Lewis R, Dixon J (2005). *NHS Market Futures: Exploring the impact of health service market reforms*. London: King's Fund.

Lewis R, Gillam S, C Jenkins (2001). *Personal Medical Services Pilots: Modernising primary care*. London: King's Fund.

London Health Planning Consortium (1981). *Primary Health Care in Inner London: Report of a study group* (Chair Donald Acheson). London: London Health Planning Consortium.

Marshall M, Harrison S (2005). 'It's about more than money: financial incentives and internal motivation'. *Quality and Safety in Health Care*, vol 14, pp 4–5.

NHS Alliance/Primary Care Report (2003). *Clinician Engagement: A national survey*. Retford: NHS Alliance.

NHS Executive (1999). *Primary Care Trusts: Establishing better services*. London: NHS Executive.

Regan E (2002). *Driving Seat or Back Seat? GPs' views on and involvement in primary care trusts*. Birmingham: Health Services Management Centre, University of Birmingham.

Saultz JW, Lochner J (2005). 'Interpersonal continuity of care and care outcomes: a critical review'. *Annals of Family Medicine*, vol 3, pp 159–66.

Smith J, Mays N, Dixon J, Goodwin N, Lewis R, McClelland S, McLeod H, Wyke S (2004). *A Review of the Effectiveness of Primary Care-led Commissioning and its Place in the NHS*. London: The Health Foundation.

Wiener J, Lewis R, Gillam S (2001). *US Managed Care and PCTs: Lessons for a small island from a lost continent*. London: King's Fund.

Linked publications

We publish a wide range of resources on health and social care. See below for a selection. For our full range of titles, visit our website at **www.kingsfund.org.uk/publications** or call Sales and Information on 020 7307 2591.

Forthcoming titles
Regulation in the New NHS Market
Jennifer Dixon

The role of regulation in a market with a variety of health care providers – including NHS foundation hospitals, privately run diagnostic and treatment centres, and potentially staff-led primary care services – is likely to be quite different to that of the regulatory system we have today. Anticipating a further statutory review of health regulation, this paper will consider how best to combine economic and quality regulation, look at whether the new market can be managed to avoid major organisational failures, and review the roles of the various stakeholders.

December 2005 ISBN 1 85717 540 9 £5.00

How Do We Deal with Failure?
Keith Palmer

One in four NHS trusts in England ended the year in deficit, the impact of the NHS reforms will be to magnify financial imbalances at a significant number of trusts, with the real risk that some of them will fail. Currently, there is no plan for dealing with failure in the NHS. This paper considers proposals for dealing with financial instability – heading off failure before it happens and proposing a regime to manage failure that cannot be averted. It emphasises the need for mechanisms not only to restore financial viability, but also to protect the quality of patient care.

December 2005 ISBN 1 85717 542 5 £5.00

Incentives in the New NHS Market

Rebecca Rosen, Anthony Harrison, Jenny Grant

While incentives to maximise productivity and reduce waiting times may be appropriate for elective care, they are less useful – and may even be deleterious – for emergency care and services for patients with long-term conditions. Here, the avoidance of hospitalisation may be a more appropriate aim, yet commissioners, primary care providers and NHS trusts do not have strong incentives to work towards this aim. This paper will consider how best to design appropriate incentives for different parts of the health care system to ensure that perverse impacts are anticipated and minimised.

January 2006 ISBN 1 85717 537 9 £5.00

Published titles

NHS Market Futures: Exploring the impact of health service market reforms

Richard Lewis, Jennifer Dixon

Despite initially rejecting the notion of an internal NHS market when it came to power in 1997, the Labour government has re-introduced competition to health services over the past three years. The market now emerging is the product of a series of separate policy developments – including extending choice of provider, expanding the role of the private sector and introducing payment by results – and consequently no one is sure what it will ultimately achieve. This paper analyses the government's market reforms, considering whether they can meet the core aims of the NHS, looking at the challenges they present, and exploring options for meeting those challenges.

September 2005 ISBN 1 85717 534 4 28 pages £5.00

An Independent Audit of the NHS Under Labour (1997–2005)
King's Fund

The Labour Party came to power in 1997 promising to 'save' the NHS. Since then it has invested unprecedented levels of funding in the health service, but has emphasised that the extra money must be linked to 'reform'. This audit, commissioned by *The Sunday Times*, assesses the Labour government's performance against its targets to bring down waiting times; recruit more health care professionals; and improve care in cancer, heart disease and mental health.

March 2005 ISBN 1 85717 488 7 88 pages £20.00

Practice-Led Commissioning: Harnessing the power of the primary care frontline
Richard Lewis

Practice-led commissioning – which involves primary care clinicians in commissioning care and services – could help meet two challenges. First, it could boost the strength of commissioning. Second, it could harness the talents of clinicians in managing and planning health services. This paper looks at the benefits of practice-led commissioning, and what it could mean within the new NHS structures. It explores the lessons of GP fundholding, total purchasing, and locality/GP commissioning pilots. Finally, it looks at ways of implementing practice-led commissioning, highlighting strategic risks and identifying where practice-led commissioning would be most welcome.

June 2004 ISBN 1 85717 506 9 32 pages £5.00

Government and the NHS: Time for a new relationship?
Steve Dewar

A range of public services, including higher education, housing, and public service broadcasting, are now being funded, delivered, or regulated through agencies working at arm's length from government. This paper looks at the conceptual and practical challenges – as well as the potential benefits – of arm's-length governance for the NHS, reviews past arguments, and considers how a new arm's-length NHS agency, accountable to Parliament, could work with government to improve health care. It argues that such an agency could make the NHS more accountable, transparent, and inclusive while also freeing up the government to consider the impact of factors such as housing and education on health.

October 2003 ISBN 1 85717 481 x 62 pages £6.50

What Is the Real Cost of More Patient Choice?
John Appleby, Anthony Harrison, Nancy Devlin

At first glance, an increase in patient choice seems to be unequivocally 'a good thing'. But what trade-offs are really involved – and what price are we prepared to pay? And how far can individual freedoms be extended while retaining the essential objectives of the NHS? This discussion paper sets out the questions that the government needs to answer if it wants to place patient choice at the heart of a health care system funded by tax-payers. These include how extra costs will be met, whether patients are willing and able to exercise choice in their own best interests, and what kinds of limits to choice might be needed.

June 2003 ISBN 1 85717 473 9 64 pages £6.50

Can Market Forces be Used for Good?
Jennifer Dixon, Julian Le Grand, Peter Smith

The government is committed to changing the NHS and making services more responsive to public demands. Meanwhile, there is ongoing debate about the benefits of market disciplines versus planned provision. This paper asks whether a highly centralised system can sit comfortably alongside a market-led approach, and whether market forces can respond effectively to demands of an ageing population. It brings together the views of three expert commentators: Julian Le Grand says stronger market incentives would improve performance among secondary care providers; Peter Smith argues against even modest experimentation with stronger market incentives; and Jennifer Dixon looks at the possibility of combining the best aspects of market disciplines with planned provision.

May 2003 ISBN 1 85717 477 1 49 pages £6.50

Future Directions for Primary Care Trusts
Richard Lewis, Jennifer Dixon, Stephen Gillam

The government has set out demanding modernisation plans for the NHS. It wants providers to be more responsive to patients, and market excesses to be curbed by better regulation and new models of social ownership. Meanwhile primary care trusts (PCTs) have been struggling to rise to the challenge. As a result, two new policy themes have emerged: stronger market incentives and decentralisation of budgetary power. This paper looks at how PCTs can adapt to these new policies and strengthen their commissioning role.

May 2003 ISBN 1 85717 513 1 16 pages £5.00